A SIMPLIFIED HIP FLEXOR EXERCISE MANAUL

Hip stretches: what to look for and how to get started

KAIN PARSONS

Table of Contents

CHAPTER ONE

Hip flexor tightness affects both men and women.

Hip stretches: what to look for and how to get started

Tight hips can be relieved with specific exercises and stretches that target the hip flexors and other muscles around the hips.

Inactivity and prolonged sitting can cause tight hips. According to the Arthritis Foundation, regular exercise is one of the best ways to keep hips flexible and pain-free.

By focusing on the hips, exercises can help:

- ensuring that the hips can move freely.

- Increasing the strength of the muscles around it

- Relieving discomfort

reducing the risk of hip injury

reduction of hip surgery in osteoarthritic individuals

Learn the best stretches for relieving hip tightness in this article. As a bonus, we also offer advice on the best way to use the foam roller.

How to perform ten hip stretches.

The following exercises will help alleviate hip tightness and protect against injury by strengthening and stretching the muscles around the hips.

Before embarking on a new exercise regimen, people should

consult with their doctor. Injuries can be avoided by beginning exercises slowly and increasing the number, length, and intensity over time.

The following are some additional tips for stretching effectively:

Pre-exercise muscle loosening can be achieved by taking a warm bath or shower.

It's important to avoid overextending yourself.

When holding stretches, allow your breath to flow freely and do not hold it in.

1. When a chair is not in use, it is

• Place a chair with its back against a wall.

It is best to sit with one's legs bent at a 90-degree angle on the edge of the seat.

• Cross your arms and rest one hand on the shoulder of the

person on the other side. Relax and recline in your chair.

Slowly rise to a standing position by leaning forward with a straight back and shoulders.

Slowly return to your seat.

• Repeat as many times as you like.

2. Lifting one's knees

1.

Lie on your back with your legs extended on the floor or a mat.

2.

The left knee should be brought up to the torso. Gently pull the knee in toward the chest with both hands.

3.

Return to the starting position after holding this stretch for 10 seconds and then repeating the exercise twice more.

4.

Repeat on the other leg. a.

5.

On each leg, do 10 repetitions of this exercise.

3. Stretching the internal hip rotator

1.

Snuggle into the back of a chair with your back against it.

2.

You can also lift your right leg and place it on your left leg with the right knee pointing outward.

3.

The right thigh can be gently pressed down with one hand until you feel a slight resistance.

4.

Maintain a straight back while slanting forward slightly at the hips to improve your posture. Exhale slowly as you do this.

CHAPTER TWO

5.

Aim for a 30-second hold of this position. You can do this again and again.

4. Hip rotator stretch on the outside

1.

Sit on a yoga mat with your legs extended and your back straight.

2.

Cross your left leg over your right leg so that your left ankle rests next to your right knee.

3.

Push your left knee toward your right shoulder with your right arm until you feel resistance. Breathe out slowly. Only go so far before you feel the pain.

4.

Aim for a 30-second hold of this position. Do the same with your other leg.

5. Rotation of the hips twice

1.

Bend the knees while lying on your back on the floor or on a mat. Take a step away from the body with your arms.

2.

Lower yourself to the floor on your left side, keeping your knees together. Make sure your thighs are parallel to your body at all times.

3.

Turn your head to the right. Hold the floor or mat tightly with both shoulders.

4.

For up to 30 seconds, keep your body in this position.

5.

As you slowly raise your knees, make a full circle with your head where it was before.

6.

Continually switch sides.

6. Stretching the hip flexors and quadriceps

1.

Position yourself in front of a wall with your feet hip-width apart, facing the wall. Place your hands on the wall to keep yourself balanced.

2.

Keep your knee bent as you take a step back with your right foot.

3.

Make a slight bend in your left knee, being careful not to let it go past your toes.

4.

Keep your buttocks tight and tucked under your hips by squeezing them. The front of your right hip and thigh should feel slightly pulled.

5.

For up to 60 seconds, hold this position.

6.

Continually switch sides.

7. flexion of the hip

1.

Position yourself in front of a wall with your feet hip-width apart, facing the wall. Place your hands on the wall to keep yourself balanced.

2.

Keep your back straight and tighten your stomach muscles.

3.

The left leg should be slowly extended behind the body. As far back as you can without letting your lower back arch, extend your leg. Take five seconds to hold this position.

4.

Repeat 10 times, returning to the beginning position each time.

5.

Attempt the exercise from the opposite side.

8. A hip abduction

1.

Face a wall and keep your feet together. Balance yourself by placing your hands on either the wall or your hips.

2.

Raise the left leg as far out to the side as you can without rotating your hips. Hold for a full 5 seconds.

3.

Repeat 10 times, returning to the beginning position each time.

4.

Attempt the exercise from the opposite side.

9. Bridge

Pin it to your Pinterest board.

1.

The best position to do this is on your back on the floor or a yoga mat. Kneel on the floor with your arms at your sides. Face the floor with your palms down.

2.

Lift the pelvis and lower back off the floor with a gentle inclination. Take five seconds to hold this position.

3.

Begin by lowering the top of your spine, then work your way down to your buttocks, and slowly return to the starting position.

4.

Repetition is encouraged up to a maximum of ten times.

CHAPTER THREE

10. Stretch your hips and back.

Pin it to your Pinterest board.

1.

On the floor or a mat, lie down on your back with your knees bent. Bend your knees.

2.

Pull the knees toward the chest with both hands.

3.

Bring the knees closer to the shoulders with each exhalation. Don't push yourself too far.

4.

Hold this position for 30 seconds after bringing the knees as close as possible to the shoulders.

Other at-home remedies for tight hips

Exercises and stretches are not the only ways to loosen tight hips; the following practices may also help:

a foam roller

Pin it to your Pinterest board.

Use a foam roller to relieve sore muscles. Sporting goods stores and online retailers carry these rollers.

Foam rollers can be used to loosen up tight hips.

1.

Make sure that the roller is placed under your body, just below your left hip.

2.

Keep the weight off of the hip by placing the forearms on the floor.

3.

Bend the knee at a 90-degree angle and move the right leg to the side.

4.

To support yourself, keep your left leg extended behind you with your toes on the floor.

5.

The left hip should be rolled over the foam roller and then back.

6.

For 30 seconds, keep doing this movement.

7.

Repeat on both sides several times per day.

Massage

Massaging the hips can help loosen the muscles in a person's body. Additionally, it aids in the breakdown of scar tissue, increases blood flow, and alleviates muscle tension and pain.

If you're having trouble getting your hands to move smoothly across your skin, try using a natural lubricant like coconut or almond oil. It is possible to buy both coconut oil and almond oil on the internet.

Heat

Muscle tension can be relieved by applying a heat pack or hot water bottle to the hip area. If necessary, repeat this treatment several times a day.

Inflammation can worsen if heat is applied to a recent injury, so avoid it at all costs. In the first 72 hours after an injury, ice should be used to reduce swelling and inflammation.

Sore muscles can be soothed with heat packs and wraps, which can be purchased at pharmacies or online.

Movement

The hip flexors are in a shortened position when sitting, which can lead to tight hips.

People with conditions like rheumatoid arthritis, a well-known cause of hip pain, may find that inactivity exacerbates their symptoms of inflammation.

In order to avoid this and loosen up tense muscles, it is recommended that people move around a lot.

Aim to move around for at least a few minutes each hour.

A high-quality bed frame

Hip pain may be alleviated or prevented by using a high-quality mattress. If you have a problem with your hips, a mattress made of foam or latex may be the best option for you.

Summary

Hip tightness and pain can be relieved most effectively through the use of specific stretches and exercises.

CHAPTER FOUR

Preventing hip injuries is easier with regular exercise.

The use of heating pads and foam rollers, two other common at-home remedies, may also help loosen up tight hips.

Even so, anyone who is suffering from severe or persistent hip pain should consult a physician so that the underlying cause may be identified and appropriate treatment may be administered.

Continued participation in activities that aggravate hip pain should be avoided. Seek out the assistance of a physical therapist or personal trainer if you feel you need it.

When and how to treat a hip flexor injury

The hip flexor muscles can be pulled, strained, torn, or injured, resulting in a hip flexor strain. The main symptom is sharp pain, which can be brought on by a variety of activities.

For example, femur bone is connected to lower back and hips and groin by hip flexor tendons. The hip flexor muscles are a group of muscles that all work together to enable movement.

Major muscles of the iliac and psoas referred to collectively as the iliopsoas

"rectus femoris" refers to the quadriceps muscle group.

Injuries, pain, and decreased mobility can all result from overusing or stretching these muscles and tendons.

Hip injuries can range in severity from minor sprains that don't necessitate medical attention to more serious fractures that cause muscles to separate from the bone. Sprains of the hip flexors that involve a break of both muscle and bone are known as third-degree sprains.

Hip flexor strain signs and symptoms

• Hip or pelvic pain that comes on suddenly and sharply after a trauma to the area

Leg ache when attempting to lift it

Upper leg muscle cramps, stiffness, and a feeling of weakness

• swelling

muscle cramps in the thighs or hamstrings

ability to kick, jump or sprint indefinitely

mobility and discomfort, such as limping, may be impaired

Exercises

The muscles in the hip flexors can be strengthened with hip exercises. Stretching at home is a great way to alleviate muscle tension and prevent further injury in the process.

Swimming and cycling can help build strength and prevent hip flexor strain in addition to at-home exercises.

Preparing your muscles for stretching by warming them up before you begin your workout can help you avoid further injury.

Heat and a few minutes of light walking are excellent ways of warming up before beginning stretching.

Hip flexor strain can be alleviated with these exercises.

The stretches listed below can help with:

- lessen the tenseness

- Allow for greater adaptability

- train your muscles to grow

- protect yourself from harm

Stretching the hip flexors

Persons need to place their hands on something solid in front of them while standing in wide walking position. Bend the front knee as you forward lunge. They should keep their back straight while pushing their hips forward. Repeat for a total of five sets of 20–30 seconds.

Butterflies stretched out on the couch

Individuals should place their soles of their feet together and bend their knees outwards while sitting upright on the floor. With their heels gently pulled inwards, they should be able to lower their knees even more toward the floor. Hold the stretch for a few minutes.

CHAPTER FIVE

With their knees bent and feet on the ground, one can perform this pose. Once their hips are off the ground, they should inhale before contracting their glutes. Continue holding for a few seconds before lowering slowly.

Lunges

To begin, a person should stand straight with their feet firmly planted on the ground. Once the hips are on the floor, they will step forward with the right foot, bending their knee and shifting their weight to that leg. The other side should then be done the same way.

The flexion of the hips

With their legs straight, people should begin lying on their backs. In order to avoid straining, they will slowly pull the knee of their right leg toward their chest. Continue on the other side by slowly lowering your leg.

Inverted hip flexion

Take a seat facing up on a bench. The bottom edge of the bench should be where the sit bones are for proper posture. To do this, stand with one foot firmly on the ground and the other leg bent and raised toward the chest. Take five deep breaths on one side, then switch. Repeat this process a total of nine times. If you feel any discomfort, you should stop right away.

What other options exist?

Some people choose to self-treat minor hip flexor injuries rather than go to the doctor.

Hip flexor strain can be treated in a number of ways.

keeping the muscles at a rest by avoiding activities that could put additional strain on them

compressing the affected area with an over-the-counter or prescription-only wrap

using an ice pack, which can be purchased in pharmacies or online, to the affected area heat packs, which can be purchased in pharmacies or online, can be applied to the afflicted area.

• a relaxing soak in the tub or shower

Aspirin, ibuprofen (Advil, Motrin), and acetaminophen (Tyleenol) are all over-the-counter pain relievers (Aleve)

It's critical to take these medications exactly as prescribed and not for longer than the recommended 10-day period.

A visit to the doctor should be made if the pain persists despite the above-mentioned remedies.

Surgery

X-rays, MRIs, and CT scans are commonly used to determine if a bone has been fractured in more serious cases.

A physical therapist or surgeon may be recommended by a doctor if the muscle damage is severe enough. However, this kind of damage is extremely uncommon.

In cases where the symptoms don't go away after a week of rest and treatment at home, it may be necessary to seek medical attention.

Temporary respite

While a mild hip flexor strain may heal within a few weeks, a more severe strain may take longer to heal.

Causes

Hip flexor strains commonly occur as a result of rapid, unusually fast muscle contractions. When a person brings their knee toward their torso, their hip flexors are activated.

Dance, martial arts, and running all put the hip flexors under the most stress. Hip flexor strains and injuries, which can tear muscles, are more common in athletes who use their hip flexors in their sport or training.

Immediately following the unexpected movement, a

person's anterior hip will typically "pop." Swelling and pain are common side effects. Many hip flexor wounds are thought to be linked to hamstring strains in sports medicine.

Preventive measures to take

Athletes and those who regularly engage in strenuous activities that could damage or overstretch the hip flexors can take preventative measures to avoid hip flexor strain.

Before engaging in any physical activity, it is important to ensure that the muscles are properly warmed up and that exercises are performed to strengthen them.

In addition, a healthy weight and a well-balanced diet can keep the body in good shape and lessen the strain on the hips.

Takeaway

As painful as hip flexor strain is, it is rarely a cause for alarm. There is a wide range in the length of time it takes to heal a strain, from a few weeks for minor injuries to up to six weeks for more serious ones.

Resting and avoiding activities that may have aggravated the injury are the best ways to speed up the healing process and ensure a quick recovery.

THE END